BORON AND TESTOSTERONE

Easy and Delicious Boron Rich Recipes with a food list designed for peak performance and male health

Dr. VICTORIA H. VINCENT

3

Chapter 1

The Science of Testosterone

Understanding Testosterone

Testosterone, often heralded as the quintessential male hormone, plays a pivotal role not just in male sexual health but in overall well-being. This hormone, produced primarily in the testes in men and smaller amounts by the ovaries in women, with some production also occurring in the adrenal glands, serves as a cornerstone for various physiological processes.

In men, testosterone's influence begins early, even before birth, guiding the development of male sex organs. As boys transition into puberty, a surge in testosterone levels brings about changes such as increased muscle mass, deeper voice, and growth of body hair. But its role extends beyond these visible markers of masculinity.

Testosterone is integral to the regulation of libido and erectile function in men. It also contributes significantly to mood regulation, bone density, and muscle strength. The hormone's effects on muscle and fat distribution are why it's closely associated with male physical appearance, including the maintenance of muscle mass and the prevention of excessive fat accumulation. Moreover, testosterone has been found to play a role in cognitive functions, including memory and concentration. It also influences emotional well-being, with low levels being linked to mood swings, irritability, and depression.

The body's testosterone levels naturally fluctuate due to various factors, including age. Typically, testosterone levels peak in early adulthood and gradually decrease with age, a decline that can lead to conditions like andropause, often referred to as male menopause, which may manifest in symptoms such as reduced libido, fatigue, and decreased bone density.

The balance of testosterone is crucial to health. Too much testosterone can lead to aggressive behaviors and an increased risk of heart disease, while too little can contribute to a lack of energy, reduced muscle mass, and osteoporosis. Thus, maintaining optimal testosterone levels is key to supporting a man's health and well-being throughout his life.

Understanding testosterone and its myriad roles underscores the importance of hormonal balance in men's health. It's not just about sexual function; testosterone's reach spans physical, mental, and emotional health, highlighting its significance well beyond its role in male puberty and virility.

Functions and Importance of Testosterone

Testosterone, a key hormone in the human body, plays a vital role in both men and women, though it is more prominent and widely recognized for its effects in males. Its functions and importance span across various physiological and psychological aspects of health.

In Men:

- **Sexual Development and Reproductive Function**: Testosterone is crucial for the development of male sexual characteristics during puberty, including the growth of the penis and testes, voice deepening, and facial and body hair. It is essential for sperm production and maintaining libido.

- **Bone Density and Muscle Strength**: This hormone helps in maintaining bone density and supports the muscular structure of the body. It influences fat distribution, contributing to a higher muscle-to-fat ratio, which is why men typically have more muscle mass and less body fat than women.

- **Mood Regulation**: Testosterone has a significant impact on mood and mental health. Adequate levels are associated with improved mood, well-being, and energy levels, whereas low levels can be linked to fatigue, depression, and irritability.

- **Cognitive Functions**: Research suggests that testosterone plays a role in certain cognitive functions, including memory and concentration. Higher testosterone levels have been associated with reduced risks of Alzheimer's disease in men.

• **Heart Health**: Testosterone influences heart health by affecting the dilation of blood vessels and aiding in the maintenance of cholesterol levels. However, the relationship between testosterone levels and heart health is complex, and both low and high levels can pose risks.

In Women:

• **Ovarian Function**: While present in much lower levels, testosterone in women is produced by the ovaries and adrenal glands and plays a role in ovarian function and bone strength. It also contributes to libido.

- **Muscle and Bone Health**: Similar to its role in men, testosterone in women contributes to muscle strength and bone density, helping prevent osteoporosis.

- **Mood and Well-being**: In women, testosterone is thought to contribute to overall mood stabilization and feelings of well-being.

Overall Importance:

Testosterone's importance extends beyond just the physical traits often associated with masculinity. It is vital for overall health and well-being, influencing a broad range of bodily functions from metabolism to mood regulation. The hormone's balance is crucial; both excessive and deficient levels can lead to health issues. For men, maintaining optimal testosterone levels is key to supporting sexual health, physical strength, cognitive function, and emotional well-being. In women, while the hormone is present in smaller amounts, it still plays a significant role in health and vitality.

Factors Influencing Testosterone Levels in Men

Testosterone levels in men are influenced by a broad array of factors ranging from physiological conditions, and lifestyle choices, to environmental exposures. Understanding these factors is crucial for managing health and well-being, as testosterone plays a pivotal role in various bodily functions, including reproductive health, muscle mass, bone density, and mood regulation.

Physiological Factors

- **Age**: Testosterone levels naturally decrease with age, typically starting to decline after the age of 30 at a rate of about 1% per year. This gradual decrease can affect muscle mass, strength, and sexual function.

- **Genetics**: Genetic factors can influence the baseline levels of testosterone, including variations in the androgen receptor gene that may affect how the body responds to testosterone.

- **Hormonal Regulation**: The hypothalamus and pituitary gland play a key role in regulating testosterone production. Any imbalance in this regulatory axis can impact testosterone levels.

Health Conditions

- **Hypogonadism**: This condition, characterized by impaired testicular function, can lead to significantly reduced testosterone production.

- **Obesity**: Excess body fat, particularly abdominal fat, can convert testosterone into estrogen, lowering testosterone levels.

- **Chronic Diseases**: Conditions like type 2 diabetes, liver or kidney disease, and hormonal disorders can negatively affect testosterone production.

- **Sleep Disorders**: Quality of sleep has a direct impact on testosterone levels, with poor sleep patterns being linked to reduced testosterone.

Lifestyle and Behavioral Factors

- **Diet**: A diet lacking in essential nutrients or high in processed foods can adversely affect testosterone levels. Certain nutrients, like vitamin D and zinc, are particularly important for maintaining optimal testosterone levels.

- **Physical Activity**: Regular exercise, especially strength training and high-intensity interval training (HIIT) can help boost testosterone levels. Conversely, excessive exercise without adequate rest can lead to decreased testosterone.

- **Stress**: Chronic stress elevates cortisol levels, which can inhibit testosterone production and overall hormonal balance.

- **Substance Use**: Alcohol and the use of certain drugs (including anabolic steroids) can significantly disrupt testosterone production and hormonal balance.

Environmental Factors

- **Exposure to Endocrine Disruptors**: Chemicals found in plastics, pesticides, and personal care products can act as endocrine disruptors, affecting testosterone levels.

- **Temperature**: Testicular temperature regulation is crucial for testosterone production. Overheating, as can occur with frequent use of saunas or hot tubs, may temporarily reduce testosterone levels.

Medical Treatments and Interventions

- **Medications**: Certain medications, including opioids, steroids, and medications used to treat prostate cancer, can impact testosterone levels.

- **Surgical Interventions**: Surgery involving the reproductive organs or hormone-producing glands can affect testosterone production.

Chapter 2

Boron Unveiled

A Mineral Overview of Boron

Boron is a fascinating trace mineral that, despite its minimal presence in the human body, plays a significant role in health and disease prevention. It's found in small amounts in the Earth's crust and various environmental sources, from soil and water to plants and foods. Boron's journey from an obscure element to a nutrient of interest in health and nutrition underscores its unique and multifaceted roles.

Physical and Chemical Properties

Boron is a metalloid, meaning it possesses properties intermediate between metals and non-metals. This characteristic makes boron incredibly versatile, contributing to its wide range of applications, from glass and ceramics manufacturing to agriculture and even as a neutron absorber in nuclear reactors. In its natural state, boron rarely exists alone and is typically found in compounds with oxygen, such as borates.

Dietary Sources

The human intake of boron is primarily through dietary sources, with fruits, vegetables, nuts, and legumes being particularly rich in boron. Foods like avocados, almonds, prunes, and chickpeas, as well as drinking water, can contribute to daily boron consumption. The boron content in these foods depends significantly on the soil's boron levels where they are grown.

The Biological Role of Boron in the Human Body

Bone Health and Development

One of the most well-documented roles of boron is in bone health. It influences the metabolism of minerals that are crucial for bone growth and maintenance, such as calcium, magnesium, and phosphorus. Boron is believed to enhance the body's ability to use these minerals effectively, thereby contributing to the prevention of bone diseases like osteoporosis. It also plays a role in regulating the hormones involved in bone health, including vitamin D and estrogen, further underscoring its importance in maintaining strong bones.

Hormonal Regulation

Boron has a notable impact on the body's hormonal balance. It affects the synthesis and activity of sex hormones, particularly estrogen and testosterone. This can have significant implications for both men and women, influencing aspects such as libido, muscle mass, and the symptoms experienced during menopause. By modulating the levels and activity of these hormones, boron contributes to overall well-being and health.

Cognitive Function

Emerging research suggests that boron is beneficial for cognitive performance. Adequate boron intake has been associated with improved brain function, including better cognitive, motor, and attention skills. It's thought that boron may play a role in supporting the brain's electrical activity and cognitive processes, although the exact mechanisms are still being explored.

Inflammatory and Antioxidant Effects

Boron exhibits anti-inflammatory and antioxidant properties, which can contribute to reducing the risk of certain chronic diseases. Inflammation is a root cause of many health conditions, including arthritis and cardiovascular disease. By mitigating inflammation and combating oxidative stress, boron can help protect against these and other health issues.

Cell Membrane Function and Signal Transduction

Boron is involved in the integrity and function of cell membranes, as well as the transmission of signals within cells. It influences various cell signaling pathways, which are essential for the body's responses to different stimuli and for maintaining homeostasis. These roles are critical for the proper functioning of cells and the overall health of tissues and organs.

Immune System Support

There is evidence to suggest that boron plays a role in supporting the immune system. While the research in this area is still developing, boron's anti-inflammatory properties, combined with its potential effects on cell signaling, may contribute to a more robust immune response.

The Connection of Boron and Hormonal Regulation

Boron plays a nuanced and influential role in the body's hormonal regulation, highlighting its importance beyond being a mere trace mineral. Its impact on hormonal health is both broad and profound, affecting various hormones that are crucial for overall well-being and physiological balance. The connection between boron and hormonal regulation encompasses several key areas:

Estrogen and Testosterone

One of the most significant effects of boron on hormonal regulation is its influence on sex hormones, particularly estrogen and testosterone. Research has shown that boron can increase the levels of these hormones in the body, which has various implications for health and disease prevention.

- **Estrogen**: Boron appears to enhance the body's use of estrogen, a hormone that plays a vital role in bone health, mood regulation, and various reproductive functions. By modulating estrogen levels, boron contributes to the maintenance of bone density and reduces the risk of osteoporosis, especially in postmenopausal women. Additionally, boron's influence on estrogen may have protective effects against hormone-related cancers.

- **Testosterone**: In men, boron supplementation has been linked to increased testosterone levels, which is essential for muscle growth, bone density, libido, and overall energy levels. By supporting natural testosterone production, boron can contribute to improved physical strength, mood stability, and sexual health.

Vitamin D

Boron's interaction with vitamin D further exemplifies its role in hormonal regulation.

Vitamin D, while often classified as a vitamin, functions similarly to a hormone and is crucial for calcium absorption and bone health. Boron is believed to enhance the body's response to vitamin D, improving calcium metabolism and contributing to stronger bones and teeth. This synergistic effect between boron and vitamin D underscores the importance of boron in maintaining skeletal health.

Insulin

Emerging evidence suggests that boron may also play a role in glucose metabolism and insulin sensitivity. Insulin is a hormone that regulates blood sugar levels, and boron's potential to influence insulin response can have implications for energy metabolism and diabetes prevention. By possibly improving insulin sensitivity, boron contributes to a more efficient regulation of blood sugar levels, which is crucial for metabolic health.

Thyroid Hormones

Although research in this area is still developing, there is interest in boron's potential effects on thyroid hormone production. The thyroid hormones play a pivotal role in regulating metabolism, energy levels, and overall metabolic rate. By influencing the activity of enzymes involved in thyroid hormone synthesis, boron may indirectly affect metabolic processes and energy balance.

Chapter 3

Boron and Testosterone Enhancement

How Boron Boosts Testosterone Levels

The relationship between boron supplementation and increased testosterone levels in men has garnered significant interest in the scientific community. Numerous studies have explored this connection, revealing how boron plays a pivotal role in modulating testosterone, a key hormone responsible for regulating muscle mass, bone density, libido, and overall energy levels. The scientific evidence supporting boron's ability to boost testosterone levels highlights its potential as a natural supplement for enhancing men's health and hormonal balance.

Mechanisms of Action

1. **Inhibition of Sex Hormone-Binding Globulin (SHBG)**: One of the primary mechanisms through which boron is thought to increase testosterone levels is by inhibiting the activity of SHBG. SHBG is a protein that binds to testosterone, rendering it inactive. By inhibiting SHBG, boron increases the concentration of free testosterone— the bioavailable form of the hormone that can actively influence physiological processes.

2. **Enhancement of Steroid Hormone Production**: Boron appears to influence the activity of enzymes involved in the steroidogenesis pathway, the process by which steroid hormones, including testosterone, are synthesized in the

body. By modulating these enzymatic activities, boron can potentially increase the natural production of testosterone.

3. **Interaction with Vitamin D and Magnesium**: Boron has been shown to improve the body's utilization of vitamin D and magnesium, nutrients that are crucial for optimal testosterone synthesis. Vitamin D, in particular, has been linked to testosterone production, and boron's ability to enhance vitamin D's effects further supports its role in boosting testosterone levels.

Supporting Studies

Several studies have provided empirical evidence supporting the role of boron in increasing testosterone levels:

- A study published in the "Journal of Trace Elements in Medicine and Biology" found that men who took a daily boron supplement of 10 mg for one week experienced significant increases in their free testosterone levels compared to baseline measurements.

- Another study highlighted that short-term boron supplementation led to an increase in total and free testosterone levels, along with a decrease in SHBG levels, suggesting that boron's effect on SHBG is a key factor in its ability to enhance testosterone levels.

Clinical Implications

The scientific evidence suggests that boron supplementation could be a viable strategy for individuals looking to naturally improve their testosterone levels, potentially benefiting those with low testosterone or those seeking to enhance muscle mass, bone health, or overall vitality. However, it's important to approach supplementation with caution, as excessive boron intake can lead to adverse effects. Optimal dosages for specific health outcomes are still being studied, and individuals should consult with healthcare providers before starting any new supplement regimen.

Boron's Influence on Hormonal Pathways

Boron's influence on hormonal pathways in the human body underscores its significance as a trace mineral with broad physiological implications. Its role extends beyond simple nutrient interactions, affecting various hormonal systems that regulate essential bodily functions. Boron's impact on hormonal pathways is complex, involving modulation of sex hormones, vitamin D metabolism, and possibly insulin and thyroid function, among others.

Sex Hormones: Estrogen and Testosterone

Boron exerts a notable effect on the metabolism of sex hormones, particularly estrogen and testosterone, which are critical for reproductive health, bone density, and muscle strength.

Several mechanisms have been proposed for boron's action:

- **Modulation of Sex Hormone-Binding Globulin (SHBG)**: Boron can influence levels of SHBG, a protein that binds to sex hormones and regulates their bioavailability. By decreasing SHBG levels, boron increases the free (active) form of estrogen and testosterone, enhancing their physiological effects.

- **Enzymatic Activity**: Boron is thought to affect the activity of enzymes involved in the synthesis and metabolism of estrogen and testosterone. This can lead to increased production or reduced breakdown of these hormones, contributing to higher circulating levels.

Vitamin D Metabolism

Boron interacts with the metabolism of vitamin D, a hormone-like compound essential for calcium absorption and bone health. By influencing vitamin D's availability and activity, boron indirectly supports bone formation and maintenance. This interaction is particularly important given the widespread issues of vitamin D deficiency and its implications for bone diseases such as osteoporosis.

Insulin Sensitivity

Emerging evidence suggests that boron may play a role in glucose metabolism and insulin sensitivity. Insulin, a hormone produced by the pancreas, is essential for regulating blood sugar levels. Boron's potential to enhance insulin sensitivity could have implications for energy utilization and the management of conditions like diabetes, although more research is needed to fully understand this relationship.

Thyroid Hormone Regulation

While research in this area is still developing, there is interest in boron's potential effects on thyroid function. The thyroid gland produces hormones that regulate metabolism, energy levels, and overall metabolic rate. Boron may influence the synthesis or activity of thyroid hormones, contributing to metabolic health, though detailed mechanisms and outcomes require further investigation.

Anti-inflammatory and Antioxidant Pathways

Boron has been shown to possess anti-inflammatory and antioxidant properties, which can influence hormonal health indirectly. Inflammation and oxidative stress can disrupt hormonal balance and signaling. By mitigating these conditions, boron may support the stability and function of hormonal pathways, contributing to overall health.

Chapter 4

Optimizing Boron Intake

A Guide to Dietary Sources

Here's a guide to dietary sources that can serve as natural supplementation of boron:

Fruits

- **Avocados**: High in boron and healthy fats, avocados are an excellent addition to any diet.
- **Apples**: A common fruit that provides a modest amount of boron alongside fiber and various vitamins.
- **Pears**: Another boron-rich fruit, pears also offer fiber and vitamin C.
- **Grapes (and raisins)**: Grapes and their dried counterparts, raisins, contain boron and antioxidants.

- **Berries**: Strawberries, raspberries, and blackberries can provide small amounts of boron.

Vegetables

- **Leafy Greens**: Spinach, kale, and Swiss chard are not only rich in vitamins and minerals but also contain boron.
- **Broccoli**: This cruciferous vegetable offers boron along with a host of other nutrients like vitamins C and K.
- **Potatoes**: Both sweet and regular potatoes are good sources of boron, vitamin C, and fiber.

Nuts and Seeds

- **Almonds**: Known for their healthy fats, almonds are also a good source of boron.
- **Hazelnuts**: Like almonds, hazelnuts offer boron and vitamin E.

- **Sunflower Seeds**: These seeds are a snackable source of boron, protein, and healthy fats.

Legumes

- **Chickpeas**: Also known as garbanzo beans, chickpeas contain boron, protein, and fiber, making them an excellent dietary choice.

- **Lentils**: High in protein and fiber, lentils also provide a good amount of boron.

- **Soybeans (and soy products like tofu)**: Soybeans are a versatile source of boron, protein, and isoflavones.

Other Sources

- **Dried Fruits**: Apart from raisins, dried apricots, prunes, and dates are concentrated sources of boron.

- **Wine and Beer**: These beverages can contain boron, likely derived from the soil in which the grapes or grains were grown. However, consumption should be moderate.

- **Coffee and Tea**: Both beverages provide trace amounts of boron, in addition to their stimulating effects.

Incorporating Boron into Your Diet

To naturally supplement boron through your diet, consider incorporating a variety of these foods into your meals. For example, starting your day with a smoothie made with berries, spinach, and almond milk can boost your boron intake. Snacking on nuts or adding chickpeas and broccoli to your salads or main dishes are other effective ways to ensure you receive this vital mineral.

Types of Boron Supplements, Dosages, and Recommendations

Understanding the types of boron supplements, recommended dosages, and general guidelines can help optimize health benefits while minimizing any potential risks.

Types of Boron Supplements

1.   **Boron Citrate**: This is a common form of boron supplement where boron is bound to citric acid. It's known for good bioavailability and is often used for bone health and to improve metabolic processes.

2.   **Boron Glycinate**: In this compound, boron is chelated with glycine, an amino acid. This form is highly bioavailable and gentle on the digestive system, making it a preferred choice for increasing boron levels effectively.

3. **Boron Aspartate**: Boron aspartate involves boron combined with aspartic acid. It's another chelated form that's easily absorbed by the body, used for similar health benefits as other forms.

4.   **Boric Acid (in supplements)**: While boric acid is more commonly known for its external uses, it's also available in some oral supplements designed for health purposes, not to be confused with its industrial or antiseptic uses.

5.   **Sodium Borate**: This form of boron is bound with sodium. It's used in some supplements and offers a way to increase boron intake, though it's less common than the other forms.

Recommended Dosages

The optimal dosage of boron varies depending on individual health goals, age, and dietary intake. In general, supplementation in the range of 3 to 10 mg per day is considered safe and potentially beneficial for adults. It's important to start with a lower dose to assess tolerance and gradually increase if needed, without exceeding the upper recommended limits.

Safety and Tolerable Upper Intake Levels

While boron is safe for most people when taken in recommended amounts, consuming high doses (above 20 mg per day) over extended periods could lead to boron toxicity. Symptoms of excessive boron intake include digestive discomfort, skin inflammation, and irritability. The specific tolerable upper intake level (UL) for boron has not been universally established, but staying within the suggested dosage range is advisable to avoid adverse effects.

Recommendations for Use

- **Consult a Healthcare Provider**: Before starting any new supplement regimen, including boron, consult with a healthcare professional to determine the most appropriate dosage for your specific health needs and to avoid interactions with other medications.

- **Assess Dietary Intake**: Consider the amount of boron you're already getting from your diet. High-boron foods may reduce the need for supplementation or allow for a lower supplemental dose.

- **Monitor Your Response**: Pay attention to how your body responds to boron supplementation, and adjust the dosage as needed, under the guidance of a healthcare provider.

- **Quality Matters**: Choose high-quality boron supplements from reputable manufacturers to ensure purity and accuracy in dosing.

Maximizing Absorption: Tips for Effective Boron Supplementation

Maximizing the absorption and effectiveness of boron supplementation involves understanding how it interacts with the body and other nutrients. Boron's bioavailability can be influenced by dietary factors, timing of intake, and the overall balance of minerals in the diet. Here are some tips to enhance the absorption and benefits of boron supplementation:

1. Combine with Magnesium and Calcium

Boron works synergistically with magnesium and calcium, two minerals essential for bone health. Incorporating adequate amounts of these minerals into your diet can enhance the effectiveness of boron, particularly for improving bone density and preventing osteoporosis. Consider a balanced intake of these minerals through diet or supplements.

2. Ensure Adequate Vitamin D Levels

Vitamin D plays a critical role in calcium absorption and bone health. Sufficient levels of vitamin D can enhance boron absorption and its beneficial effects on the skeletal system. Sun exposure, vitamin D-rich foods, and supplements are ways to ensure adequate vitamin D levels.

3. Maintain a Balanced Diet

A well-rounded diet rich in fruits, vegetables, nuts, and whole grains provides not only dietary boron but also other nutrients that work in concert with boron. This nutritional balance supports overall health and optimizes the body's use of boron.

4. Pay Attention to Timing

Taking boron supplements at certain times can maximize absorption. For instance, taking boron with meals can improve its uptake, as food can increase stomach acidity, enhancing mineral absorption. Avoiding high-fiber meals when taking boron supplements may also aid absorption since fiber can bind to minerals and reduce their bioavailability.

5. Stay Hydrated

Adequate hydration supports overall metabolic processes, including the digestion and absorption of nutrients. Drinking plenty of water throughout the day can help ensure that boron and other supplements are effectively processed by the body.

6. Limit Alcohol and Caffeine

Alcohol and caffeine can interfere with the body's ability to absorb minerals, including boron. Moderating the intake of these substances can help improve the overall effectiveness of boron supplementation.

7. Consider Supplement Form

The form of boron supplement can affect its bioavailability. Boron citrate, glycinate, and aspartate are among the well-absorbed forms. Choosing a high-quality supplement from a reputable manufacturer can also ensure that you're getting a form of boron that your body can effectively use.

8. Monitor and Adjust Based on Response

Individual responses to boron supplementation can vary. Monitoring how your body reacts and adjusting your intake (with the guidance of a healthcare provider) can help find the optimal dosage for your specific health needs.

9. Regular Blood Tests

For those taking boron supplements for specific health conditions, regular blood tests can help monitor boron levels and ensure they are within a healthy range. This can also help adjust supplementation to avoid potential toxicity.

Chapter 5

Beyond Testosterone

Bone Health and Density Improvements

Bone health and density are critical aspects of overall health, influencing not only physical strength and mobility but also affecting the risk of osteoporosis and fractures, especially as individuals age. Improving and maintaining bone health involves a multifaceted approach that includes adequate nutrition, regular physical activity, and lifestyle modifications. Here's how these elements contribute to stronger bones and improved bone density:

Nutrition for Bone Health

1. **Calcium**: This mineral is essential for bone formation and maintenance. Adequate calcium intake through dairy

products, leafy greens, fortified foods, or supplements is crucial for bone strength.

2. **Vitamin D**: Vitamin D enhances calcium absorption in the gut and is necessary for proper bone growth and remodeling. It can be obtained from sunlight exposure, fatty fish, fortified foods, and supplements.

3. **Magnesium and Potassium**: These minerals contribute to bone health by supporting bone density. Nuts, seeds, whole grains, and bananas are good sources.

4. **Vitamin K**: Important for bone metabolism and the regulation of calcium in bones and other tissues. Leafy green vegetables like kale and spinach are excellent sources.

5. **Protein**: Adequate protein intake is essential for healthy bones. Sources

include lean meats, dairy products, legumes, and nuts.

6. **Boron**: This trace mineral supports calcium and magnesium use in the body and influences estrogen and vitamin D levels in the blood, all of which are important for maintaining healthy bones.

Physical Activity

1. **Weight-Bearing Exercises**: Activities that force you to work against gravity, such as walking, jogging, and climbing stairs, help build and maintain bone density.

2. **Strength Training**: Lifting weights or using resistance bands can stimulate bone growth and reduce the risk of osteoporosis.

3. **Balance and Flexibility Exercises**: Practices like yoga and Tai Chi can

improve balance, reduce the risk of falls, and maintain bone health.

Lifestyle Modifications

1. **Limiting Alcohol Consumption**: Excessive alcohol can interfere with the balance of calcium and the production of hormones, which are vital for bone health.

2. **Quitting Smoking**: Smoking can reduce bone density and increase the risk of fractures by interfering with the body's ability to absorb calcium.

3. **Maintaining a Healthy Weight**: Being underweight increases the risk of bone loss and fractures while being overweight can put additional stress on the bones.

Monitoring Bone Health

1. **Regular Screenings**: Bone density tests can help diagnose osteoporosis

before a fracture occurs and monitor the effectiveness of treatment if you're taking medication for bone health.

2. **Supplements**: If dietary intake is insufficient, supplements may be necessary to meet the daily requirements for bone health nutrients, especially calcium, vitamin D, and magnesium.

Cognitive Function and Mental Clarity

Cognitive function and mental clarity are essential aspects of overall health and well-being, affecting our ability to think, learn, remember, and make decisions. These cognitive processes are influenced by a variety of factors, including nutrition, physical activity, mental stimulation, and lifestyle habits. Understanding how to support and enhance cognitive function can lead to improved productivity, a sharper mind, and a reduced risk of cognitive decline with age.

Nutrition for Cognitive Health

1. **Omega-3 Fatty Acids**: Found in fatty fish (like salmon, mackerel, and sardines), flaxseeds, and walnuts, omega-3s are crucial for brain health, supporting neuron function and reducing inflammation.

2. **Antioxidants**: Vitamins C and E, flavonoids, and carotenoids act as antioxidants, protecting brain cells from damage. Berries, nuts, dark chocolate, and green leafy vegetables are rich in antioxidants.

3. **B Vitamins**: B6, B12, and folic acid help reduce homocysteine levels in the blood, which, in high levels, is

linked to cognitive decline. Sources include whole grains, meat, eggs, and dairy.

4. **Boron**: This trace mineral plays a role in brain function and mental clarity. Foods rich in boron, such as nuts, fruits, and leafy greens, can support cognitive health.

Physical Activity and Brain Health

1. **Aerobic Exercise**: Activities like walking, jogging, swimming, and cycling increase heart rate and blood flow to the brain, enhancing neurogenesis (the creation of new neurons) and improving memory and thinking skills.

2. **Strength Training**: In addition to physical benefits, resistance training has been shown to improve

executive function, memory, and cognitive flexibility.

3. **Mind-Body Exercises**: Yoga and Tai Chi not only improve physical fitness but also benefit mental health, reducing stress and anxiety, which can cloud cognitive function.

Mental Stimulation

1. **Continuous Learning**: Engaging in new activities, learning new skills, or pursuing hobbies stimulates the brain and can improve cognitive function.

2. **Puzzles and Brain Games**: Activities that challenge the brain, such as crossword puzzles, Sudoku, and strategy games, can help keep the mind sharp and improve problem-solving skills.

3. **Reading and Writing**: Regularly engaging in reading and writing

activities can enhance vocabulary, comprehension, and critical thinking skills.

Lifestyle Habits for Cognitive Clarity

1. **Adequate Sleep**: Quality sleep is crucial for cognitive function. During sleep, the brain consolidates memories and clears out toxins, supporting mental clarity.

2. **Stress Management**: Chronic stress can impair cognitive function. Techniques such as meditation, deep breathing exercises, and mindfulness can help manage stress levels.

3. **Social Interaction**: Maintaining strong social connections and engaging in meaningful conversations can stimulate cognitive processes and reduce the risk of cognitive decline.

4. **Limiting Alcohol and Avoiding Smoking**: Excessive alcohol consumption and smoking can negatively impact brain health, reducing cognitive function and increasing the risk of dementia.

Immune System Support and Inflammation Reduction

Supporting the immune system and reducing inflammation is pivotal for maintaining overall health and preventing chronic diseases. The immune system acts as the body's defense mechanism against infections and diseases, while inflammation is a natural response to injury or infection. However, chronic inflammation can lead to various health issues, including autoimmune diseases, heart disease, and cancer.

Here's how nutrition, lifestyle choices, and other factors can play a role in bolstering immune function and mitigating inflammation:

Nutrition for Immune Support and Inflammation Reduction

1. **Antioxidant-Rich Foods**: Antioxidants combat oxidative stress and reduce inflammation. Foods high in vitamins C and E, selenium, and flavonoids, such as berries, nuts, green leafy vegetables, and citrus fruits, are excellent choices.

2. **Omega-3 Fatty Acids**: These fats have potent anti-inflammatory properties. Sources include fatty fish (salmon, mackerel, sardines), flaxseeds, chia seeds, and walnuts.

3. **Probiotics and Prebiotics**: A healthy gut microbiome is crucial for immune function. Probiotics (found in yogurt, kefir, and fermented foods) and prebiotics (found in garlic, onions, and bananas) support gut health.

4. **Whole Grains and Fiber**: High-fiber foods and whole grains help reduce inflammatory markers. They also support gut health, which is closely linked to immune function.

5. **Boron**: As a trace mineral, boron has been shown to influence the body's use of other minerals and vitamins, potentially supporting immune health and reducing inflammation.

Physical Activity

Moderate, regular exercise boosts the immune system and can help reduce inflammation. Activities like brisk walking, cycling, and swimming, when done consistently, can have a positive impact on immune health and help lower inflammation levels.

Stress Management

Chronic stress can weaken the immune system and contribute to inflammation. Techniques such as mindfulness meditation, yoga, deep breathing exercises, and ensuring adequate sleep can help manage stress and support immune function.

Adequate Sleep

Sleep is crucial for immune health. Lack of sleep can impair the production of cytokines, a type of protein that targets infection and inflammation, effectively reducing the body's immune response.

Hydration

Staying well-hydrated assists in the production of lymph, a fluid that circulates white blood cells and nutrients throughout the body, supporting the immune system.

Limiting Alcohol and Quitting Smoking

Excessive alcohol consumption and smoking can impair immune function and exacerbate inflammation. Reducing alcohol intake and quitting smoking are beneficial for boosting immune health and reducing inflammation.

Regular Health Check-ups

Regular medical check-ups can help identify and address potential health issues that may impact immune function or contribute to chronic inflammation.

Chapter 6

Implementing Boron into Your Wellness Routine

Daily Boron Requirements

Boron is an essential trace mineral with a range of biological functions, contributing to bone health, cognitive performance, and hormonal balance, among others. However, because Boron does not have a formally established Recommended Daily Allowance (RDA), tailoring your intake to meet your specific health needs and conditions can be nuanced. The amount of boron considered beneficial can vary based on dietary sources, individual health status, and specific health goals.

General Guidelines on Boron Intake

While there is no official RDA for boron, various studies and health organizations suggest that adults can safely consume between 1 to 3 milligrams (mg) of boron per day through their diet to support general health. Some research indicates that doses up to 10 mg per day can offer specific health benefits without causing adverse effects. It's important to note that the optimal intake might vary depending on individual factors such as age, sex, and health conditions.

Factors Influencing Boron Requirements

1. **Dietary Patterns**: People consuming a diet rich in fruits, vegetables, nuts, and legumes are likely to have higher boron intakes due to the natural boron content of these foods.

Individuals with dietary restrictions or those consuming a limited variety of foods might need to pay more attention to their boron intake.

2. **Health Goals**: Specific health objectives can influence boron needs. For example, higher intakes (around 3-10 mg per day) might support bone health, improve wound healing, or aid in hormonal balance.

3. **Age and Gender**: While detailed guidelines for different age groups and genders are not established, the physiological demands and hormonal profiles can influence optimal boron intake. For instance, postmenopausal women or older adults concerned about bone health may benefit from ensuring adequate boron intake.

4. **Geographical Location**: The boron content in soil can vary greatly by region, affecting the boron levels in plant-based foods. Individuals in areas with low soil boron might have lower dietary intake and may need to be more mindful of their boron sources.

Tailoring Your Boron Intake

1. **Evaluate Dietary Sources**: Assess your regular diet to estimate your daily boron intake. Include boron-rich foods like avocados, nuts, dried fruits, and leafy greens to naturally increase your intake.

2. **Consider Supplementation**: If dietary sources are insufficient or if you have specific health goals that might benefit from higher boron intake, consider supplements. Always start

with lower doses to assess tolerance and avoid exceeding 20 mg per day, as higher intakes could lead to toxicity.

3. **Monitor Health Changes**: Pay attention to any changes in your health or symptoms that might indicate either a deficiency or an excess of boron. Adjust your intake accordingly and consult with a healthcare provider for personalized advice.

4. **Consult With a Healthcare Provider**: Before starting any new supplement regimen, including boron, it's advisable to consult with a healthcare professional. They can provide guidance based on your health status, dietary habits, and specific needs.

Foods and Vitamins That Complement Boron

1.   **Magnesium**: Magnesium plays a vital role in bone health and metabolic functions. Boron and magnesium work together to strengthen bones and improve calcium utilization. Foods rich in magnesium include spinach, almonds, black beans, and avocado.

2.   **Calcium**: Essential for bone health, calcium absorption, and utilization can be enhanced by boron. This synergy is crucial for preventing osteoporosis and maintaining healthy bone structure. Dairy products, fortified plant milks, kale, and broccoli are excellent sources of calcium.

3.   **Vitamin D**: Vitamin D is necessary for calcium absorption and bone health. Boron is believed to assist in the metabolism of vitamin D, enhancing its

effects on calcium metabolism and bone density. Fatty fish, egg yolks, fortified foods, and sensible sun exposure can increase vitamin D levels.

4. **Phosphorus**: Like calcium, phosphorus is important for bone health. Boron works with phosphorus to maintain and repair bones and teeth. Foods high in phosphorus include salmon, yogurt, turkey, and lentils.

5. **Vitamin C**: Known for its role in immune function and collagen synthesis, vitamin C also contributes to bone matrix formation. Boron and vitamin C together can support bone regeneration and overall skeletal health. Citrus fruits, strawberries, bell peppers, and kiwi are rich in vitamin C.

6. **Silicon**: Silicon is another trace mineral that benefits bone and

connective tissue health. The combination of boron and silicon can further support bone formation and maintenance. Sources of silicon include bananas, green beans, whole grains, and beer.

7. **Omega-3 Fatty Acids**: Omega-3s have anti-inflammatory properties that can be beneficial for conditions like arthritis, where boron also plays a role. Eating foods rich in omega-3s, such as salmon, flaxseeds, and walnuts, can complement the anti-inflammatory effects of boron.

Implementing Synergistic Nutrition

To maximize the synergistic effects of boron with other nutrients, consider incorporating a variety of these foods into your daily diet. For example, a salad made with leafy greens (magnesium), topped with salmon (omega-3s and vitamin D), and a side of yogurt (calcium and phosphorus), can provide a nutrient-rich meal that supports bone health and overall wellness.

Exercise Recommendation to Enhance Boron Efficacy

To enhance the efficacy of boron, particularly in its roles supporting bone health, hormonal balance, and cognitive functions, incorporating a tailored exercise regimen can be highly beneficial. Exercise not only improves overall health but also amplifies the biological activities of boron in the body. Here's a deeper look into how specific types of exercises can complement boron supplementation:

Weight-Bearing Exercises

Weight-bearing exercises are activities that make you move against gravity while staying upright, thereby strengthening bones and muscles through the force exerted on them. These exercises are crucial for stimulating bone formation and preventing bone loss, aligning perfectly with boron's role in enhancing bone density and health.

Examples: Walking, jogging, stair climbing, dancing, and playing sports like tennis or basketball.

Mechanism: The stress placed on bones during weight-bearing activities prompts bone-forming cells to build new bone tissue, enhancing bone strength and density. Boron contributes to this process by improving the body's use of calcium, magnesium, and vitamin D—key nutrients for bone health.

Strength Training

Strength or resistance training involves the use of weights, resistance bands, or body weight to build muscle and strength. This type of exercise not only supports muscular development but also has a positive impact on bone health, complementing boron's effects.

Examples: Lifting weights, using resistance bands, bodyweight exercises (like push-ups and squats), and machine-based exercises.

Mechanism: Strength training increases muscle mass, which in turn places a higher demand on bones, leading to increased bone density. Boron aids in this process by supporting testosterone levels, which is important for muscle growth and recovery, thereby enhancing the benefits of strength training on the body.

Flexibility and Balance Workouts

Exercises focusing on flexibility and balance are essential for maintaining joint health, preventing falls, and reducing stress levels. These exercises support the body's overall well-being and can enhance the mental health benefits of boron.

Examples: Yoga, Tai Chi, Pilates, and stretching routines.

Mechanism: Such practices improve joint mobility, reduce the risk of injuries, and lower stress levels through mindful movements and breathing techniques. Boron's role in reducing inflammation and supporting cognitive functions, such as focus and mental clarity, is complemented by the stress-reducing and cognitive-enhancing benefits of flexibility and balance workouts.

Aerobic Exercises

Aerobic exercises improve cardiovascular health and endurance, promoting blood circulation and oxygen flow throughout the body, including to the brain and bones.

Examples: Swimming, cycling, brisk walking, and aerobic classes.

Mechanism: Enhanced blood flow increases nutrient delivery to tissues, including boron, improving its bioavailability and function in the body. This type of exercise also supports hormonal balance and can help mitigate stress, aligning with Boron's systemic benefits.

Practical Tips for Incorporating Exercise

1.   **Consistency is Key**: Regular exercise maximizes the health benefits of boron. Aim for at least 150 minutes of moderate aerobic activity or 75 minutes of vigorous

activity per week, along with muscle-strengthening activities on two or more days per week, as recommended by health guidelines.

2. **Diversify Your Routine**: Incorporating a mix of weight-bearing, strength training, flexibility, and aerobic exercises can provide comprehensive health benefits and enhance boron's efficacy.

3. **Listen to Your Body**: Tailor your exercise intensity and duration to your fitness level and health status. Adjust as needed to avoid injury and ensure sustainable practices.

Chapter 7

Safety and Side Effects

Understanding the Safe Use of Boron

Here's a comprehensive guide to navigating the safe use of boron, including recommended dosages, potential side effects, and contraindications.

Recommended Dosages

The optimal dosage of boron varies based on individual needs, age, and health status. For adults, a daily intake of 1 to 3 milligrams (mg) from all sources (dietary and supplemental) is generally considered sufficient to support health without causing adverse effects. Some studies suggest that doses up to 10 mg per day can be beneficial for specific health outcomes, such as improving bone density or hormonal balance, but these should be approached with caution and under professional guidance.

Potential Side Effects

While boron is safe for most people when consumed in amounts within the recommended dosage, excessive intake can lead to side effects, including:

- **Gastrointestinal discomfort**: Nausea, diarrhea, and vomiting can occur with high doses of boron.
- **Dermatological reactions**: Skin irritation, rashes, or inflammation may arise from excessive boron exposure.
- **Neurological symptoms**: High levels of boron intake have been associated with headaches, lethargy, and a lack of coordination in some cases.

It's important to note that the risk of experiencing these side effects increases significantly with doses exceeding 20 mg per day.

Contraindications

Certain individuals should exercise caution or avoid boron supplementation altogether:

- **Pregnant and breastfeeding women**: The safe use of boron has not been well established in pregnant or breastfeeding women. It's advisable to stick to dietary sources of boron and avoid supplementation unless directed by a healthcare provider.

- **Individuals with hormone-sensitive conditions**: Since boron can affect hormone levels, including estrogen and testosterone, individuals with hormone-sensitive conditions (such as breast, ovarian, or prostate cancers) should consult a healthcare professional before using boron supplements.

- **People with kidney issues**: Boron is excreted through the kidneys. Individuals with kidney disease or impaired kidney function should be cautious with boron intake, as their bodies may not efficiently eliminate excess boron, increasing the risk of toxicity.

Monitoring and Adjusting Boron Intake

- **Dietary assessment**: Regularly assess your diet to estimate your boron intake. Foods like nuts, fruits, vegetables, and legumes are natural sources of boron. Adjust your dietary intake or supplementation based on this assessment.

- **Listen to your body**: Pay attention to any adverse symptoms that may arise from boron supplementation and adjust your intake accordingly.

- **Consult with healthcare professionals**: Before starting any boron supplement, especially if you have existing health conditions or are taking medications, it's crucial to consult with a healthcare provider. They can offer guidance on safe dosages and monitor for potential interactions with medications or other supplements.

Potential Side Effects and How to Mitigate Them

While boron is essential for health, benefiting bone density, hormonal balance, and cognitive function, exceeding recommended dosages can lead to potential side effects. Understanding these side effects and how to mitigate them is crucial for safely incorporating boron into your health regimen.

Potential Side Effects of Excessive Boron Intake

1. **Gastrointestinal Issues**: High doses of boron can cause nausea, vomiting, diarrhea, and general gastrointestinal discomfort.

2. **Dermatological Reactions**: Excessive boron intake might lead to skin irritation, rash, or other dermatological issues.

3. **Neurological Symptoms**: Overconsumption of boron has been associated with headaches, fatigue, tremors, and confusion in some cases.

4. **Hormonal Imbalance**: Given boron's role in hormone regulation, excessively high levels could potentially disrupt hormonal balance, affecting estrogen and testosterone levels.

Mitigation Strategies

1. **Adhere to Recommended Dosages**: The most effective way to mitigate side effects is to adhere to the recommended dosages of boron. For adults, this typically ranges from 1 to 3 mg per day through diet, with some studies suggesting up to 10 mg per day from supplements can be safe under guidance. Avoid exceeding these amounts to minimize risk.

2. **Monitor Intake from All Sources**: Consider both dietary sources and supplements when calculating your

total daily boron intake. Foods such as nuts, legumes, fruits, and vegetables contribute to your overall intake.

3. **Stay Hydrated**: Drinking plenty of water can help mitigate gastrointestinal side effects by aiding digestion and facilitating the excretion of excess boron.

4. **Discontinue Use if Symptoms Occur**: If you experience adverse effects after starting boron supplementation, discontinue use and consult a healthcare provider. They can help determine if symptoms are related to boron intake and advise on further action.

5. **Consult Healthcare Providers Before Supplementation**: Before adding boron supplements to your regimen,

especially if you have existing health conditions or are on medication, consult a healthcare professional. They can provide personalized advice based on your health status.

6. **Gradual Introduction**: When starting boron supplementation, consider gradually introducing the supplement to your routine to assess tolerance and minimize potential side effects.

7. **Regular Health Check-ups**: Regular check-ups can help monitor the impact of boron supplementation on your health, allowing for adjustments as needed based on professional advice.

8. **Consideration for At-Risk Populations**: Pregnant or breastfeeding women, individuals with kidney disease, and

those with hormone-sensitive conditions should exercise caution with boron supplementation, adhering strictly to advised dosages or avoiding supplementation altogether.

Chapter 8:

Boron-Rich Recipes for Boosting Testosterone Levels

Avocado and Citrus Salad

Ingredients:

- 2 ripe avocados, sliced

- 1 orange, peeled and segments

- 1 grapefruit, peeled and segments

- A handful of arugula or mixed greens

- 2 tablespoons olive oil

- 1 tablespoon lemon juice

- Salt and pepper to taste

- A sprinkle of chopped walnuts

Instructions:

1. In a large bowl, combine the sliced avocados, orange segments, grapefruit segments, and mixed greens.

2. In a small bowl, whisk together olive oil, lemon juice, salt, and pepper.

3. Pour the dressing over the salad and gently toss to coat.

4. Garnish with chopped walnuts before serving.

Nutritional Information (approximate per serving):

- Calories: 250

- Protein: 3g

- Fat: 20g

- Carbohydrates: 20g

- Dietary Fiber: 7g

- Boron: Estimated 1.5mg

Broccoli and Almond Stir-Fry

Ingredients:

- 2 cups broccoli florets

- 1/2 cup almonds, sliced

- 2 tablespoons sesame oil

- 2 garlic cloves, minced

- 1 tablespoon soy sauce

- 1 teaspoon honey

- Salt and pepper to taste

Instructions:

1. Heat the sesame oil in a large pan over medium heat.

2. Add the minced garlic and sauté for 1 minute until fragrant.

3. Add the broccoli florets and stir-fry for about 5 minutes, or until they start to soften.

4. Add the sliced almonds, soy sauce, and honey. Stir well to combine and cook for another 2 minutes.

5. Season with salt and pepper to taste and serve hot.

Nutritional Information (approximate per serving):

- Calories: 220

- Protein: 6g

- Fat: 18g

- Carbohydrates: 12g

- Dietary Fiber: 4g

- Boron: Estimated 2mg

Nutty Banana Smoothie

Ingredients:

- 1 banana

- 1/4 cup walnuts

- 1 cup almond milk

- 1 tablespoon chia seeds

- A dash of cinnamon

Instructions:

1. Combine the banana, walnuts, almond milk, chia seeds, and cinnamon in a blender.

2. Blend until smooth.

3. Serve immediately, optionally garnished with a sprinkle of cinnamon on top.

Nutritional Information (approximate per serving):

- Calories: 300

- Protein: 5g

- Fat: 16g

- Carbohydrates: 36g

- Dietary Fiber: 6g

- Boron: Estimated 1mg

Quinoa and Black Bean Salad

Ingredients:

- 1 cup cooked quinoa

- 1 can black beans, rinsed and drained

- 1 avocado, diced

- 1 cup cherry tomatoes, halved

- 1/2 cup corn (fresh or frozen and thawed)

- 1/4 cup red onion, finely chopped

- 1/4 cup cilantro, chopped

- 2 tablespoons olive oil

- Juice of 1 lime

- Salt and pepper to taste

Instructions:

1. In a large bowl, combine cooked quinoa, black beans, diced avocado, cherry tomatoes, corn, red onion, and cilantro.

2. In a small bowl, whisk together olive oil, lime juice, salt, and pepper to create the dressing.

3. Pour the dressing over the salad and toss gently to combine.

4. Adjust seasoning with salt and pepper as needed. Serve chilled or at room temperature.

Nutritional Information (approximate per serving):

- Calories: 320

- Protein: 10g

- Fat: 14g

- Carbohydrates: 42g

- Dietary Fiber: 10g

- Boron: Estimated 1mg

Baked Salmon with Walnut Crust

Ingredients:

- 4 salmon fillets (about 6 ounces each)

- 1/2 cup walnuts, finely chopped

- 2 tablespoons Dijon mustard

- 2 tablespoons honey

- Salt and pepper to taste

- Lemon wedges for serving

Instructions:

1. Preheat your oven to 375°F (190°C). Line a baking sheet with parchment paper.

2. In a small bowl, mix the walnuts, Dijon mustard, and honey.

3. Season the salmon fillets with salt and pepper. Place them on the prepared baking sheet.

4. Spread the walnut mixture over the top of each salmon fillet.

5. Bake in the preheated oven for 12-15 minutes, or until the salmon is cooked through and the crust is golden.

6. Serve hot with lemon wedges on the side.

Nutritional Information (approximate per serving):

- Calories: 400

- Protein: 35g

- Fat: 24g

- Carbohydrates: 12g

- Dietary Fiber: 2g

- Boron: Estimated 0.8mg

Spinach and Almond Feta Salad

Ingredients:

- 4 cups spinach leaves, washed and dried

- 1/2 cup crumbled feta cheese

- 1/4 cup sliced almonds, toasted

- 1/4 cup dried cranberries

- 2 tablespoons balsamic vinegar

- 3 tablespoons olive oil

- Salt and pepper to taste

Instructions:

1. In a large salad bowl, combine the spinach, feta cheese, toasted almonds, and dried cranberries.

2. In a small bowl, whisk together balsamic vinegar, olive oil, salt, and pepper to create the dressing.

3. Drizzle the dressing over the salad and toss gently to combine.

4. Serve immediately, adjusting seasoning with salt and pepper as needed.

Nutritional Information (approximate per serving):

- Calories: 220

- Protein: 6g

- Fat: 18g

- Carbohydrates: 12g

- Dietary Fiber: 3g

- Boron: Estimated 0.9mg

Turkey and Quinoa Stuffed Peppers

Ingredients:

- 4 large bell peppers, halved and seeds removed

- 1 pound ground turkey

- 1 cup cooked quinoa

- 1 can (15 oz) black beans, drained and rinsed

- 1 cup corn (fresh or frozen)

- 1 cup tomato sauce

- 1 teaspoon cumin

- 1 teaspoon chili powder

- 1/2 teaspoon garlic powder

- Salt and pepper to taste

- 1/2 cup shredded cheese (optional)

- Fresh cilantro for garnish

Instructions:

1. Preheat oven to 375°F (190°C).

2. In a skillet over medium heat, cook the ground turkey until browned. Drain any excess fat.

3. Stir in the cooked quinoa, black beans, corn, tomato sauce, cumin, chili powder, garlic powder, salt, and pepper. Cook for another 5 minutes until everything is well combined and heated through.

4. Arrange the bell pepper halves in a baking dish, cut side up. Spoon the turkey and quinoa mixture into each bell pepper half.

5. Cover the baking dish with aluminum foil and bake for 30 minutes. Remove the foil, top with shredded cheese if using, and bake for another 10

minutes or until the cheese is melted and the peppers are tender.

6. Garnish with fresh cilantro before serving.

Nutritional Information (approximate per serving):

- Calories: 350

- Protein: 25g

- Fat: 10g

- Carbohydrates: 45g

- Dietary Fiber: 8g

- Boron: Estimated 0.5mg

Apple and Walnut Oatmeal

Ingredients:

- 1 cup rolled oats

- 2 cups almond milk

- 1 apple, diced

- 1/4 cup walnuts, chopped

- 1 teaspoon cinnamon

- 1 tablespoon honey or maple syrup

Instructions:

1. In a medium saucepan, bring the almond milk to a boil. Add the rolled oats and reduce the heat to a simmer.

2. Cook the oats, stirring occasionally, for about 5 minutes until they are soft and have absorbed most of the almond milk.

3. Stir in the diced apple, chopped walnuts, cinnamon, and honey or maple syrup. Cook for another 2 minutes.

4. Serve hot, with additional almond milk or toppings if desired.

Nutritional Information (approximate per serving):

- Calories: 300

- Protein: 8g

- Fat: 12g

- Carbohydrates: 44g

- Dietary Fiber: 6g

- Boron: Estimated 1.2mg

Spinach and Mushroom Egg Bake

Ingredients:

- 6 eggs

- 2 cups fresh spinach, chopped

- 1 cup mushrooms, sliced

- 1/2 cup milk (any kind)

- 1/2 cup cheese, grated (optional)

- Salt and pepper to taste

- 1 teaspoon olive oil

Instructions:

1. Preheat the oven to 375°F (190°C). Grease a baking dish with olive oil.

2. In a skillet over medium heat, sauté the mushrooms until they are soft and have released their moisture, about 5 minutes. Add the spinach and cook until just wilted.

3. In a bowl, whisk together the eggs, milk, salt, and pepper.

4. Layer the sautéed mushrooms and spinach in the bottom of the

prepared baking dish. Pour the egg mixture over the vegetables. Sprinkle with cheese if using.

5. Bake for 25-30 minutes, or until the eggs are set and the top is lightly golden.

6. Let cool for a few minutes before slicing and serving.

Nutritional Information (approximate per serving):

- Calories: 200

- Protein: 14g

- Fat: 14g

- Carbohydrates: 4g

- Dietary Fiber: 1g

- Boron: Estimated 0.4mg

Almond Butter and Banana Pancakes

Ingredients:

- 1 cup whole wheat flour

- 1 tablespoon baking powder

- 1/4 teaspoon salt

- 1 banana, mashed

- 1 cup almond milk

- 2 tablespoons almond butter

- 1 tablespoon honey or maple syrup

- 1 teaspoon vanilla extract

Instructions:

1. In a large bowl, whisk together the whole wheat flour, baking powder, and salt.

2. In another bowl, mix the mashed banana, almond milk, almond butter,

honey (or maple syrup), and vanilla extract until smooth.

3. Pour the wet ingredients into the dry ingredients and stir until just combined. Let the batter sit for 5 minutes.

4. Heat a non-stick skillet over medium heat and lightly grease it with cooking spray or oil. Pour 1/4 cup of batter for each pancake and cook until bubbles form on the surface, then flip and cook until golden brown.

5. Serve warm with additional almond butter or maple syrup.

Nutritional Information (approximate per serving):

- Calories: 280

- Protein: 8g

- Fat: 10g

- Carbohydrates: 40g

- Dietary Fiber: 6g

- Boron: Estimated 0.7mg

Lentil and Walnut Veggie Burgers

Ingredients:

- 1 cup cooked lentils

- 1/2 cup walnuts, finely chopped

- 1/2 cup breadcrumbs

- 1 egg, beaten

- 1/2 cup grated carrots

- 1/4 cup finely chopped onion

- 2 garlic cloves, minced

- 1 teaspoon cumin

- Salt and pepper to taste

- 2 tablespoons olive oil for cooking

Instructions:

1. In a large bowl, mash the cooked lentils until mostly smooth. Stir in the walnuts, breadcrumbs, beaten egg, grated carrots, onion, garlic, cumin, salt, and pepper until well combined.

2. Form the mixture into patties.

3. Heat the olive oil in a skillet over medium heat. Cook the patties for about 4-5 minutes on each side, until they are golden brown and firm.

4. Serve the veggie burgers on buns with your favorite toppings.

Nutritional Information (approximate per serving):

- Calories: 320

- Protein: 14g

- Fat: 18g

- Carbohydrates: 28g

- Dietary Fiber: 7g

- Boron: Estimated 0.8mg

Chicken and Broccoli Stir-Fry with Almonds

Ingredients:

- 1 pound chicken breast, thinly sliced

- 2 cups broccoli florets

- 1/2 cup sliced almonds

- 2 tablespoons olive oil

- 2 garlic cloves, minced

- 1 tablespoon soy sauce

- 1 tablespoon honey

- 1 teaspoon ginger, grated

- Salt and pepper to taste

- Cooked rice or quinoa, for serving

Instructions:

1. Heat 1 tablespoon of olive oil in a large skillet over medium-high heat. Add the chicken slices, season with salt and pepper, and cook until browned and cooked through. Remove from the skillet and set aside.

2. In the same skillet, add the remaining tablespoon of olive oil and the broccoli florets. Stir-fry for about 3-4 minutes until they are bright green and slightly tender.

3. Add the minced garlic and grated ginger to the skillet and cook for another minute until fragrant.

4. Return the cooked chicken to the skillet. Add the soy sauce, honey, and sliced almonds. Stir well to combine and cook for another 2-3 minutes, until everything is heated through and coated in the sauce.

5. Serve the stir-fry over cooked rice or quinoa.

Nutritional Information (approximate per serving):

- Calories: 350

- Protein: 30g

- Fat: 18g

- Carbohydrates: 18g

- Dietary Fiber: 4g

- Boron: Estimated 0.6mg

Roasted Beet and Goat Cheese Salad

Ingredients:

- 3 medium beets, peeled and diced

- 1 tablespoon olive oil

- Salt and pepper to taste

- 4 cups mixed greens (e.g., arugula, spinach, kale)

- 1/2 cup goat cheese, crumbled

- 1/4 cup pecans, toasted

- 2 tablespoons balsamic vinegar

- 1 tablespoon honey

- 1 teaspoon Dijon mustard

Instructions:

1. Preheat the oven to 400°F (200°C). Toss the diced beets with olive oil, salt, and pepper. Spread them on a baking sheet and roast for 25-30 minutes, until tender and slightly caramelized.

2. In a large salad bowl, combine the mixed greens, roasted beets, crumbled goat cheese, and toasted pecans.

3. In a small bowl, whisk together the balsamic vinegar, honey, and Dijon mustard. Drizzle the dressing over the salad and gently toss to combine.

4. Serve immediately, enjoying the blend of sweet, earthy, and tangy flavors.

Nutritional Information (approximate per serving):

- Calories: 280

- Protein: 8g

- Fat: 18g

- Carbohydrates: 22g

- Dietary Fiber: 5g

- Boron: Estimated 0.5mg

Sweet Potato and Black Bean Tacos

Ingredients:

- 2 medium sweet potatoes, peeled and diced

- 1 tablespoon olive oil

- 1 teaspoon chili powder

- Salt and pepper to taste

- 1 can (15 oz) black beans, drained and rinsed

- 8 small corn tortillas

- 1 avocado, sliced

- 1/4 cup red onion, finely chopped

- 1/4 cup fresh cilantro, chopped

- Lime wedges for serving

Instructions:

1. Preheat the oven to 425°F (220°C). Toss the diced sweet potatoes with olive oil, chili powder, salt, and pepper. Spread them on a baking sheet and roast for 20-25 minutes, until tender and lightly browned.

2. Warm the black beans in a saucepan over medium heat, seasoned with a little salt and pepper.

3. Warm the corn tortillas in the oven or on a skillet.

4. Assemble the tacos by layering the roasted sweet potatoes and black beans onto the tortillas. Top with avocado slices, chopped red onion, and cilantro.

5. Serve with lime wedges on the side for squeezing over the tacos.

Nutritional Information (approximate per serving):

- Calories: 320

- Protein: 9g

- Fat: 10g

- Carbohydrates: 50g

- Dietary Fiber: 12g

- Boron: Estimated 0.6mg

Pear and Gorgonzola Pizza with Arugula

Ingredients:

- 1 pre-made pizza dough or flatbread

- 1 pear, thinly sliced

- 1/2 cup gorgonzola cheese, crumbled

- 2 cups arugula

- 1 tablespoon olive oil

- 1 tablespoon balsamic glaze

- Salt and pepper to taste

Instructions:

1. Preheat your oven according to the pizza dough instructions. Roll out the dough on a baking sheet.

2. Arrange the pear slices evenly over the dough, and sprinkle with gorgonzola cheese.

3. Bake according to the dough's instructions, until the crust is golden and the cheese is melted and bubbly.

4. Toss the arugula with olive oil, salt, and pepper. Once the pizza is done, top it with the fresh arugula and drizzle with balsamic glaze.

5. Slice and serve immediately, enjoying the unique combination of sweet pear, tangy cheese, and peppery arugula.

Nutritional Information (approximate per serving):

- Calories: 400

- Protein: 12g

- Fat: 20g

- Carbohydrates: 45g

- Dietary Fiber: 3g

- Boron: Estimated 0.4mg

Chickpea and Avocado Wrap

Ingredients:

- 1 ripe avocado, mashed

- 1 cup cooked chickpeas

- 1/2 red bell pepper, finely diced

- 1/4 red onion, finely diced

- Juice of 1 lime

- Salt and pepper to taste

- 2 tablespoons fresh cilantro, chopped

- 2 large whole wheat tortillas

- 1 cup spinach leaves

Instructions:

1. In a bowl, combine the mashed avocado, chickpeas, diced bell pepper, onion, lime juice, salt, pepper, and cilantro. Mix well to combine.

2. Lay out the whole wheat tortillas and spread half of the avocado and chickpea mixture onto each tortilla.

3. Add a layer of spinach leaves on top of the mixture.

4. Roll up the tortillas tightly, cut them in half, and serve immediately.

Nutritional Information (approximate per serving):

- Calories: 350

- Protein: 10g

- Fat: 15g

- Carbohydrates: 45g

- Dietary Fiber: 12g

- Boron: Estimated 1mg

Baked Cod with Almond Crust

Ingredients:

- 4 cod fillets (about 6 ounces each)

- 1/2 cup almonds, finely chopped

- 1/4 cup whole wheat breadcrumbs

- 2 tablespoons olive oil

- 1 garlic clove, minced

- Zest of 1 lemon

- Salt and pepper to taste

- Lemon wedges for serving

Instructions:

1. Preheat the oven to 400°F (200°C). Line a baking sheet with parchment paper.

2. In a bowl, mix the chopped almonds, breadcrumbs, olive oil, minced garlic, lemon zest, salt, and pepper.

3. Place the cod fillets on the prepared baking sheet. Press the almond mixture onto the top of each fillet to form a crust.

4. Bake for 12-15 minutes, or until the fish flakes easily with a fork and the crust is golden.

5. Serve with lemon wedges on the side.

Nutritional Information (approximate per serving):

- Calories: 280

- Protein: 27g

- Fat: 15g

- Carbohydrates: 9g

- Dietary Fiber: 2g

- Boron: Estimated 0.5mg

Quinoa and Roasted Vegetable Salad

Ingredients:

- 1 cup quinoa, rinsed

- 2 cups water

- 1 small zucchini, diced

- 1 small yellow squash, diced

- 1 red bell pepper, diced

- 1 tablespoon olive oil

- Salt and pepper to taste

- 1/4 cup dried cranberries

- 1/4 cup pumpkin seeds

- Dressing: 2 tablespoons olive oil, 1 tablespoon lemon juice, 1 teaspoon honey, salt, and pepper

Instructions:

1. Preheat the oven to 425°F (220°C). Toss the diced zucchini, squash, and bell pepper with olive oil, salt, and pepper. Spread the vegetables on a baking sheet and roast for 20 minutes, until tender and slightly caramelized.

2. Meanwhile, bring 2 cups of water to a boil in a pot. Add the quinoa,

reduce heat to low, cover, and simmer for 15 minutes, or until all water is absorbed. Remove from heat and let it sit, covered, for 5 minutes. Fluff with a fork.

3. In a large bowl, combine the cooked quinoa, roasted vegetables, dried cranberries, and pumpkin seeds.

4. Whisk together the dressing ingredients and pour over the salad. Toss to combine.

5. Serve warm or at room temperature.

Nutritional Information (approximate per serving):

- Calories: 320

- Protein: 10g

- Fat: 14g

- Carbohydrates: 42g

- Dietary Fiber: 7g

- Boron: Estimated 0.7mg

Chapter 9

Conclusion

In conclusion, the relationship between boron supplementation and testosterone levels is a promising area of nutritional science that warrants attention for its potential health benefits. Current research indicates that boron plays a significant role in the metabolism of steroid hormones, including the natural elevation of testosterone levels, which is crucial for maintaining and improving muscle mass, bone density, cognitive function, and overall well-being.

The inclusion of boron-rich foods such as nuts, fruits, vegetables, and legumes into one's diet presents a natural, effective, and enjoyable strategy to potentially enhance testosterone levels alongside numerous other health benefits. These foods, as demonstrated through various recipes, not only offer a direct route to boron supplementation but also provide a wide array of essential nutrients that support a holistic approach to health and wellness.

For individuals looking to optimize their testosterone levels and general health, incorporating boron through dietary sources is a practical and beneficial approach. However, it's important to remember that dietary changes should be considered as part of a comprehensive lifestyle strategy that includes regular exercise, adequate sleep, and stress management for optimal hormonal balance and health outcomes.

Given the complexity of human physiology and the variability in individual responses to dietary supplements, further research is necessary to fully understand the extent of boron's benefits. As with any supplement or dietary modification aimed at achieving specific health outcomes, consultation with healthcare professionals is advisable to tailor personal health strategies to individual needs, ensuring both safety and effectiveness.

In summary, boron's potential to positively influence testosterone levels and promote better health outcomes offers an exciting avenue for nutritional intervention. By making informed choices about diet and lifestyle, individuals can harness the benefits of boron, among other nutrients, to support their health goals in a balanced and sustainable manner.

9 798879 504835